PENGUIN BOOKS

healing and cleansing with

herbal
tea

PENELOPE SACH

healing and cleansing with

herbal
tea

PENGUIN BOOKS

Penguin Books

Published by the Penguin Group
Penguin Books Australia Ltd
250 Camberwell Road
Camberwell, Victoria 3124, Australia
Penguin Books Ltd
80 Strand, London WC2R 0RL, England
Penguin Putnam Inc.
375 Hudson Street, New York, New York 10014, USA
Penguin Books, a division of Pearson Canada
10 Alcorn Avenue, Toronto, Ontario, Canada, M4V 3B2
Penguin Books (N.Z.) Ltd
Cnr Rosedale and Airborne Roads, Albany, Auckland, New Zealand
Penguin Books (South Africa) (Pty) Ltd
24 Sturdee Avenue, Rosebank, Johannesburg 2196, South Africa
Penguin Books India (P) Ltd
11, Community Centre, Panchsheel Park, New Delhi 110 017, India

First published as *The Healing Effects of Herbal Tea* by Penguin Books Australia Ltd 2000
This edition published 2003

1 3 5 7 9 10 8 6 4 2

Copyright © Penelope Sach 2000

The moral right of the author has been asserted

Cover design by Melissa Fraser, Penguin Design Studio
Text design by Ellie Exarchos, Penguin Design Studio
Typeset in 10/14.25 Legacy Serif by Post Pre-press Group, Brisbane, Queensland
Printed and bound in Australia by McPherson's Printing Group, Maryborough, Victoria

National Library of Australia
Cataloguing-in-Publication data:

Sach, Penelope.
Healing and cleansing with herbal tea.

Bibliography.
Includes index.
ISBN 0 14 300145 0.

1. Herbal teas – Therapeutic use. 2. Herbal teas. I. Title.

615.321

www.penguin.com.au

To find out more about Penelope Sach teas, visit the author at her web site on
www.penelopesach.com.au

contents

acknowledgements

This book has been a great pleasure to write, not only because I love plant medicine but also because I have the pleasure to work with exceptionally talented and professional people, several of whom I would like to thank.

Firstly, thank you to Julie Gibbs, Executive Publisher at Penguin Books, an inspiration and a great supporter of ideas. Secondly, I would like to thank Helen Pace, my dedicated and talented editor, for her gentle but precise understanding and great attention to detail. Thirdly, thanks to my writing assistant, Catherine Hanger, whose ability to see the shape through the maze is exceptional.

I would also like to thank those in Mediherb and Health World for their professional attitude to the developments in herbal medicine in Australia and globally.

Lastly, I thank my family, friends and staff who encourage me to express my ideas and give me continual support in all that I do.

preface

My philosophy is that when it comes to health and wellbeing, the simplest things in life are not only the most enjoyable and easy to pursue, but are often also the ones that achieve the greatest results.

In over fourteen years of clinical experience as a practitioner of naturopathic and herbal medicine, I have found the most common cause of illness and fatigue to be a lack of what we in the western world often take for granted – water, one of life's simplest gifts. When I confronted my clients with this basic truth many years ago, their responses were always the same: plain water is boring.

This concerned me. Knowing how vital it is to regularly drink quality fluids and, naturally, aware of the benefits of herbs, I set about researching herbal teas. It was my hope that herbal teas would encourage people to drink more, and in so doing to help themselves to better health. I developed a range of organic herbal teas called simply Herbal Teas by Penelope Sach (see next page). While they eventually went on to be served in restaurants and five-star hotels, they were initially used with my clients, especially business people trying to wean themselves off caffeine. I spoke widely about the healing effects of herbal tea and I wrote a book, *On Tea and Healthy Living*, which highlighted the importance of drinking water and other quality fluids, and which showcased a variety of herbal teas.

Thankfully, most people are now aware of the need to drink fluids, and herbal teas are more widely accepted and enjoyed. But there is still much to be said about the *quality* of herbal teas. One can't expect to enjoy the health-giving benefits of herbal tea from a teabag, which contains leaves that have been ground to a powder and hence have lost much of their healing properties. (Flavours and preservatives are then added to restore taste and colour.) Only loose, organic herbal tea without preservatives and additives can give you the healing benefits you seek and which I discuss in this book.

Healing and Cleansing with Herbal Tea is a celebration

of herbs and fine-quality herbal teas, and a guide to the creative ways of incorporating them into your lifestyle. It is my hope that even more people will seek the best quality herbal teas available, and will discover for themselves the rich flavours and the healing potential unique to herbal teas.

I make reference to these teas throughout this book. Below is a list of the teas and their ingredients.

❧ APRES: contains chamomile, fennel, peppermint, spearmint and aniseed. Used to treat insomnia or any sleeping disorder, including nightmares. Excellent for those who suffer from anxiety and stress, Apres also alleviates bad digestion, heartburn and colic in children.

❧ BERRY: contains hawthorn berry, elderberry and juniper. This tea is high in antioxidants. It boosts energy and vitality and stimulates blood circulation and the heart. I call this my 'red wine' antioxidant tea because of its sweet, strong, full taste – but of course there is no alcohol.

ᴥ LEMON TANG: contains lemongrass and peppermint. A wonderful tea to take for a hangover. It also has a calming effect on mild nervousness. Lemon Tang acts as a diuretic, and therefore alleviates fluid retention and bad digestion.

ᴥ PETAL: contains red clover, lavender, lemongrass, rose hip, rose petals and chamomile. This tea cleanses the skin and detoxifies the body. It has a very calming effect and can be used to counteract stress.

ᴥ SUMMER DELIGHT: contains peppermint, lemon thyme, calendula and spearmint. This tea is very effective in clearing the upper respiratory passages and alleviating allergies, sinus and headaches. Summer Delight is an uplifting, feel-good tea that adds clarity to a tired, overworked brain!

ᴥ TRIPLE E: contains liquorice, peppermint and fennel. Very effective in the treatment of acid stomach, bronchial conditions and arthritis. This tea boosts energy and stimulates a sluggish liver and bowel. It is also excellent for sports people. Triple E has a sweet taste, which appeals to those with a sweet tooth.

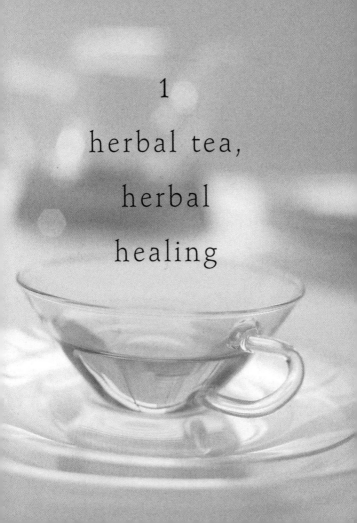

1
herbal tea,
herbal
healing

Tea has a long history as a health-giving drink. Traditionally regarded as a cure-all, tea relieved sufferers from lethargy, colds and headaches; it aided digestion; it preserved youthful skin; and it improved both the body's immunity and its longevity.

Some of these health claims have been expanded over the years, and many of you would have your own experiences of the healing effects of tea – of the way it can soothe and relax while at the same time awaken and invigorate. However, recent scientific interest in tea suggests that tea's healing potential is far more significant.

This interest in tea has focused on its disease-fighting potential; more specifically on substances called polyphenols and their antioxidant properties. Much of the research has concentrated on green tea, although herbalists know that many herbal teas also contain specific antioxidant properties.

Antioxidants and tea

The word antioxidant is used widely by scientists and the health and beauty industry, but it is important to understand exactly what we mean by this term when used in relation to tea and herbal medicine.

Let's start with oxygen. Oxygen is vital to life;

without it we cannot live. However, in giving us life oxygen paradoxically causes damage to the cell tissue in our bodies. This is called oxidation: oxygen combines with other elements and molecules in the environment to create what are called 'free radicals'. Free radicals then attack molecules in the body causing deterioration.

With the increase in pollution, pesticides, herbicides, preservatives, carbon monoxide and metals in our environment, the level of free radical activity increases. The effects of stress and an unhealthy diet also contribute to this increased activity. The free radicals cause tissue damage, which manifests as cancers, tumours, hardening of the arteries and accelerated ageing of the skin and internal organs.

Antioxidants are naturally occurring substances in plants, fresh fruit and vegetables and red wine that have the ability to combine with and neutralise free radicals to slow down or even reverse the damaging effects of oxidation. Vitamins A, E and C are antioxidants, as are many active substances in plant foods including polyphenols, which are found in a concentrated form in green tea. (I will discuss the antioxidant properties of green tea in the next chapter.) Other important antioxidants contained in tea are flavonoids, which are found in hawthorn berry tea and the tannin of black tea.

ANTIOXIDANTS ARE VITAL FOR GOOD HEALTH BECAUSE THEY:

- *neutralise free radicals to retard or slow down the ageing process*
- *assist in preventing cholesterol build-up in arteries (atherosclerosis) and making blood less prone to clotting (thus reducing the risk of thrombosis)*
- *assist in minimising the inflammation of cell tissues particularly associated with surgery*
- *assist in scavenging free radicals responsible for hangovers.*

Some plants containing antioxidants are particularly suited to herbal teas, such as hawthorn berry, grapeseed (which is utilised for support in varicose veins and capillary fragility) and cats claw (used for the immune system), all of which contain polyphenols. Herbs that contain high levels of antioxidants include turmeric (a traditional Indian herb used in arthritis and cardiovascular problems), gingko (used for circulatory problems and known for assisting memory), chaparral, Schisandra, St Mary's thistle (for more details on these three herbs see following section), ginger, rosemary and sage. Not all of these herbs translate into pleasant-tasting teas, but they can be easily blended or disguised with non-antioxidant herbs that have other therapeutic effects, such as peppermint or lemongrass. There is also a wide range of herbs that can be taken in a non-tea form such as a tablet. (A herbalist would be able to give you a full appraisal.)

It has been suggested that an antioxidant intake derived from a range of sources provides the best protection against free radicals. This, coupled with recent research proposing that tea has comparatively greater ability to disable free radicals than vegetables, would suggest that teas with antioxidant properties are an especially important element in a healthy diet.

Three important teas to protect against toxic poisoning

As we enter the twenty-first century we are subjected to increasing levels of pollution in the environment and in our food. Chaparral, Schisandra and St Mary's thistle have a very important place in modern healing because these herbs treat ailments related to toxic poisoning.

Due to its extensive content of antioxidant lignans, *chaparral* has been traditionally and now scientifically used for its anti-cancer treatments and blood-purifying properties.

The berries of the *Schisandra* vine have been used in Chinese medicine for many centuries and now with findings of its antioxidant properties this herb will take its rightful place as a key plant for the next century. Its use in treating chronic fatigue and in protecting the liver as well as its anti-depressant effects rank it as a must to incorporate as a tea (it also has quite a pleasant taste). In my clinical work I find it useful for treating those who suffer from hepatitis and for those who are withdrawing from drugs of any kind, including recreational.

The antioxidant effect of flavonolignans, known collectively as silymarin, have made *St Mary's thistle* famous in herbal medicine for its astonishing protective effects against liver toxicity. Those who have been exposed to toxins such as carbon tetrachloride, galactosamine, ethanol, paracetamol, heavy metals and drug medication can gain great benefits by regularly ingesting tea or capsules of this herb. Travellers exposed to hepatitis, alcoholic liver damage and viral infections should consider drinking this tea. For those who suffer from food intolerance, nausea or chronic constipation, St Mary's thistle mixed with liquorice, chamomile and peppermint is an excellent combination.

Health and herbal tea

One of the most attractive qualities of herbal tea is that it can be made to taste. For this reason alone tea is one of the best methods available to a herbalist for treating patients. No-one likes to swallow something that is unpleasant, even if it is good for them.

The art is in the blending. While peppermint, chamomile and lemongrass teas are delicious, some teas can be bland or even bitter when taken alone. In such cases, a good herbalist will be able to blend the required tea with another to mask and improve the taste. In most instances, teas can be blended so that their effect is synergistic. In herbal medicine this means that each ingredient works well in partnership to create a mix that is both flavoursome and therapeutic.

For example, sage tea has exceptional qualities and I often prescribe it for menopausal women. However, the taste of sage tea on its own is bitter and disagreeable. For this reason, I combine sage with lemongrass, which makes the flavour pleasant. In addition, the lemongrass helps to rid the body of excess fluid, a problem that menopausal women often report.

Herbal tea is only effective as a treatment if the active properties of the plant can be accessed by the addition of boiling water, but not all herbs release their active ingredients in this way. For example, chamomile tea is a very good treatment for anxiety, insomnia and other nervous complaints. St John's Wort has similar properties, but this plant is not readily active when combined with water. This is why St John's Wort is better taken as a tablet or tincture. A tincture is an alcohol-based solution, which carries the active properties of the herb in a concentrated form.

One of the reasons why I often favour herbal tea over other treatments is that it is easy to digest, simple to prepare and extremely safe. Tea is effortless. Even resistant patients are usually quite amenable to adding a few cups of tea to their diet. Herbal tea does not interfere with lifestyle; in fact, it enhances it because it improves health with minimal interference. And while some patients avoid tablets because they find them difficult to digest, herbal tea is likely to improve digestion, if only because it automatically increases fluid intake.

In my years as a herbalist I have noted that patients will consistently name as their favourite the tea containing ingredients their body most needs. Many patients suffering from stress and fatigue will naturally gravitate to my Triple E tea for its energising properties. Triple E is also often sought by patients who suffer sugar cravings because the inclusion of liquorice gives the tea a sweet flavour. Berry tea is a favourite of older people who enjoy the rich, satisfying flavour of this tea, which more closely approximates a traditional cup of black tea than other herbal teas with their more delicate flavours. Berry tea is also an excellent tonic for joint and circulation problems, which are common to older folk.

The average herbal tea drinker can safely consume three to eight cups of herbal tea a day. However, if you have been prescribed a special tea to treat an ailment, then you must check with your practitioner exactly how much tea you are required to take. In this case, the herbal tea is being used as a specific treatment and the instructions you are given as to its use should be followed as carefully as a prescription.

Detoxifying with herbal tea

Herbal teas play a role in detoxifying the body. The tissue in our body needs to be bathed in adequate water for cell regeneration and a healthy metabolism. This fluid also allows the toxic by-products of all bodily processes to be carried away and flushed out. This is how the body works under normal conditions. Remember that if you are not looking after your diet, are neglecting to exercise and are ingesting too much alcohol or fat, then you will be increasing the toxic waste in your body – possibly to overload.

I like to describe the working system of the body to my clients with a powerful analogy – the waterfall. A waterfall is a beautiful natural site of pure fresh running water. The clarity and purity of this water strikes us; it invites us to drink. On the other hand, a still stagnant pool choked with algae and weeds repels us. It suggests ill health and disease; it is an unclean, unhappy site.

We can visualise our bloodstream as a waterfall, constantly being renewed by fresh fluid. Our body's cells and tissues are being bathed continually and toxins swept away.

In this healthy body, the skin breathes and is clear, kidneys don't have a chance to make kidney stones, the liver detoxifies efficiently, joints are cushioned with fluid and, most obviously, the body enjoys a feeling of wellbeing and its vitality is increased.

Herbal tea – water with the addition of a medicinal plant – will offer your body dual health benefits: it will actively work to heal your body's ailments while it simultaneously detoxifies your body by bathing and nourishing the bloodstream.

Quality tea, quality healing

One critical factor determining the healing effects of herbal tea is its quality. While there are many varieties and flavours available on the market, only high-quality teas will have true therapeutic benefits.

Harvesting herbs for tea is one factor influencing the quality of the tea. The best teas are made from herbs that have been carefully picked to maintain their healing properties. For example, leafy herbs such as mint and lemongrass are ideally picked in the early morning when the dew has dried and just before the plant comes into flower. This is when the volatile oils in the leaves are at their highest concentration. Scissors or sharp shears are used to cut the herbs; breaking the stems or pulling at leaves will bruise and damage them.

Flowers and petals (in chamomile tea, for example) should be collected when the flower is fully opened. Sage is best harvested when the earliest buds appear; seeds such as fennel and dill in the autumn;

berries when the fruit is ripe and the colour at its richest. The most favourable time to harvest roots for herbal teas is in the autumn when the leaves are shed. It is during this period that the medicinal properties are most concentrated in the part of the plant that constitutes the root system.

COLLECTING HERBS

There are a number of traditional, time-honoured rituals for collecting herbs. It is said that the vital essences of herbs are at their strongest around the time of the full moon. Herbalists of old liked to collect their ingredients just as the sun came up, never in the full heat of the day.

When I first became a herbalist, I made my own teas by drying herbs in a special oven with the heat reaching not more than thirty-four degrees Celsius and with the door slightly ajar to let moisture escape. Herbs heated in severe heat or direct sunlight will lose colour and the quality of the essential oils will be depleted. The aim of drying herbs is to remove the water content only and to preserve the active ingredients. Good ventilation is essential; for this reason, herbs are often dried on racks in dark or shaded locations or hung in bunches from roof rafters to dry. Good commercial teas are dried in a variety of ways in commercial ovens; all of them based on removing moisture without removing the tea's essential qualities. Herbs should then be stored in airtight jars or containers in a cool environment.

Loose-leaf, organic teas are far and away the best choice for quality herbal healing. Organic tea that has been grown without pesticides and then naturally dried without the addition of preservatives, colours and flavours will have a much stronger therapeutic effect than highly processed teas. Good quality loose-leaf tea can also be used up to three times, which means that the effects are magnified. I usually suggest to my patients that they make up a pot of the prescribed tea and add two lots of water to it before discarding the leaves.

Processing and over-treating the plant will reduce its effectiveness. For example, organic, loose-leaf chamomile complete with flowers and a powerful natural fragrance will perform much more effectively than a single teabag full of crushed chamomile leaves that have lost much of their value in the processing and preparation. The strong scent of organic, loose-leaf tea indicates the presence of natural oils, which contain much of the plant's health-giving properties. (I will discuss this in more detail in chapter 5.) Many of these natural oils are lost in the process of crushing the leaves. In addition, a teabag does not usually contain enough tea to effect real therapeutic change. Weighing in at less than two grams, tea bags do not contain enough plant matter to allow the healing properties to work efficiently.

I firmly believe that herbal teas can heal a range of ailments and help promote all-round good health. If you have a specific problem, see a herbalist and follow directions carefully. If you already have a serious illness or disease for which you have sought medical advice, ask a herbalist to prescribe a complementary course of herbs that you can safely take in conjunction with the medical treatment. Remember, tea complements a healthy lifestyle, a lifestyle that includes regular exercise, a diet low in fat and salt but high in fibre, and adequate rest and recreation. Only then can tea realise its true healing potential.

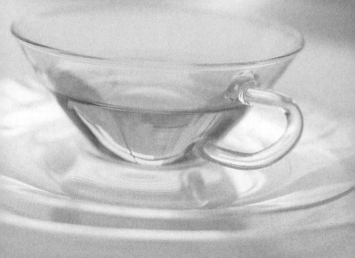

2

black and

green teas

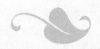

When you think of herbal teas, chances are you think of delicate teas with delicate interesting names, the kind of teas you're looking to explore further in this book. But did you know that your everyday black teas, and green teas, are also herbal teas?

Herbs are plants valued for their flavour, scent or medicinal properties and teas are simply infusions of leaves, flowers and other parts of these plants in boiling water. It follows, then, that black and green teas, which are cultivated from the same bush known as *Camellia sinensis* and are later served steeped in boiling water, are indeed herbal teas. The difference between these teas and the 'conventional' herbal teas that I write about in this book, is the presence of caffeine.

Apart from the herb kola, conventional herbal teas do not contain caffeine. Black and green teas do, albeit in varying quantities. Caffeine is actually a vital natural component of black and green teas, acting as a mild stimulant and increasing the activity of digestive juices. However the effects of caffeine are not as sharply felt in tea drinkers as they are in coffee drinkers, largely because certain properties in tea slow down the rate of caffeine absorption. The result is that the effects of caffeine are experienced more slowly but are present in the body for a longer period. This explains why tea is often described as refreshing and relaxing, yet uplifting.

HISTORICAL HEALTH CLAIMS FOR BLACK AND GREEN TEA:

- *detoxifies the body*
- *assists digestion*
- *stimulates blood flow*
- *induces clear thinking*
- *promotes longevity*
- *combats tiredness*
- *increases immunity.*

The cultivation and processing of black and green teas

Camellia sinensis, the tea bush from which black and green teas are produced, is cultivated in over thirty countries including India, Sri Lanka and China. It is best grown in high-altitude areas that enjoy warm, but rainy, conditions. After three to five years' growth, the bush is then pruned and tended and may go on to produce tea leaves for up to fifty years thereafter.

Tea leaves may be mechanically harvested, but are mostly hand plucked. Harvesting by hand ensures a higher quality tea as the 'flush' of the tea plant – the fragile new growth on a pruned plant comprising two leaves and a bud – can be carefully selected. The flush is said to produce the best tea and has a greater content of the antioxidant polyphenols.

When cultivated, the tea leaves are ready for processing. It is at this stage that the three most common types of tea are produced: green tea, black tea and oolong tea. While originating from the same tea plant, these three varieties are quite different in colour, aroma and taste.

The variety of tea undergoing the least amount of processing is *green tea*. After the leaves have been harvested, they are allowed to dry and are then heat-treated to prevent the absorption of oxygen. No further processing is required, which ensures precious antioxidants remain intact. The resulting tea has a light astringent taste and is pale light-green or yellow in colour. (Decaffeinated green tea is available for those concerned about their caffeine intake.) Green tea accounts for about twenty per cent of the world's tea production.

Black tea undergoes further processing. After drying, the tea leaves are rolled in order to release certain chemicals responsible for black tea's characteristic colour and flavour. The leaves, still greenish at this stage, are then rested and allowed to absorb oxygen (this is called oxidation or fermentation) before they are fired. The firing process is designed to halt decomposition and gives the leaves their distinctive black-tea aroma and dark-brown colour. Black tea accounts for about seventy-five per cent of the world's tea production.

Oolong tea is an exotic speciality tea produced in China and Taiwan. The process is similar to that of black tea, only the individual processing stages are much shorter. Also, in the production of oolong tea, the leaves are kept whole and are not broken by rolling. Oolong tea is like a blend of green and black teas in taste and colour. It accounts for about only five per cent of the world's tea production.

A STORY ABOUT THE ORIGINS OF TEA

In 2737 BC, the Chinese Emperor Shen Nung observed that people who boiled their drinking water were healthier than those who drank the impurities in unboiled water, so he took up this practice himself. It is believed that while the Emperor was boiling some water, leaves from the Camellia sinensis *plant fell into his pot. He drank this brew and found it to be refreshing and flavoursome.*

Antioxidants in black and green teas

Now that you know a little about the processing of tea, you'll understand more about antioxidants in black and green teas. I spoke about antioxidants in conventional herbal teas in the previous chapter. You'll recall that antioxidants are naturally occurring substances found in teas, fresh fruit and vegetables and red wine that help protect the body by neutralising harmful free radicals. Free radicals contribute to many diseases and are a cause of accelerated ageing.

All black and green tea varieties contain polyphenols, which are powerful antioxidants. The difference in the antioxidant content in each of the tea varieties is directly related to the way in which the tea is processed. I'll start with green tea, simply because it illustrates this point most effectively.

As you saw above, the production of green tea involves the least amount of processing. After being harvested, the tea leaves require only an initial drying and subsequent light heat-treatment. The absence of the oxidation or fermentation process ensures the antioxidants in green tea remain virtually unharmed. And as antioxidants are vital to the prevention of disease, ill health and ageing, which are in part caused by oxidation, green tea appears to have significant healing potential.

As black tea undergoes more rigorous processing that includes oxidation, it inevitably loses some of its antioxidant properties. However the news is not bad for black-tea drinkers. Given the high level of its consumption in the western world, black tea does markedly impact upon the antioxidant intake of individual diets. And, as antioxidants are more effective when consumed from a range of sources, teas – regardless of variety – are a necessary inclusion in one's daily diet.

More about green tea

There have been a number of amazing claims made about the therapeutic effects of green tea. You may have read about green tea's alleged link to cancer prevention and its apparent cardio-protective qualities that can help the heart resist cardiovascular diseases. It is said green tea can also promote dental health by preventing dental cavities and gingivitis. Welcome findings indeed, although there is still much research to be done in this area.

Even before green tea became the subject of research, it was known that the antioxidant polyphenols were the source of tea's health-giving potential. It made sense that green tea, which has the highest polyphenol content of all the teas, would have the greatest impact on health. (Other active ingredients in green tea are small amounts of caffeine and nutrients, as well as hundreds of aromatic oils.) Early scientific studies have discovered a range of healing effects, from the prevention of tumours to a reduction in the risk of cancer, stroke and heart attack.

SOME FINDINGS ON THE HEALING EFFECTS OF GREEN TEA:

- *lowers total cholesterol levels*
- *decreases the risk of cancer and stroke*
- *reduces blood pressure*
- *promotes longevity*
- *protects against dental cavities and gingivitis.*

Research into the healing potential of green tea continues, and while the findings are indeed remarkable, it must be remembered that green tea will only have healing effects if it is quality loose-leaf tea and when it is taken in therapeutic quantities prescribed by a herbalist.

OXALATE LEVELS IN BLACK AND GREEN TEAS

Recent research has indicated a link between kidney stones and the consumption of black tea without milk. Black tea has a high oxalate concentration (the vast majority of kidney stones are composed primarily of calcium oxalate).

Green tea contains similar levels of oxalate to black tea, but because it is brewed weaker, it yields lower oxalate concentrations.

The oxalate content of herbal teas (and coffee) can be up to thirty-two times less than that of black tea. For those who tend to form kidney stones, herbal teas make a great alternative to black tea.

3

herbs for

wellbeing

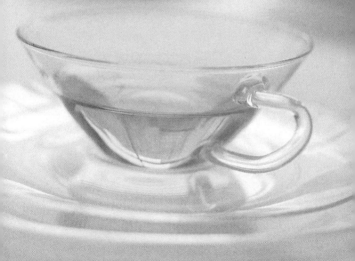

Throughout my years as a herbalist and naturopath I have been involved in hundreds of cases that illustrate how herbal teas have a positive impact on health and wellbeing. In my practice I see all kinds of people with all kinds of ailments. The most common ailments include stress, skin disorders, colds and flu, fatigue, allergies, headaches, respiratory and circulatory problems, digestive disorders, hormonal imbalances – the list is long. Herbal teas are useful in treating every one of these conditions. But before I list the most common ailments and provide some examples of how they can be treated with herbal tea, I want to explain briefly how herbs work to heal the body.

Specific herbs target specific parts of the body; for example, chamomile helps to heal disorders of the nervous system, while ginger works on the circulatory and cardiovascular systems. Some herbs, such as red clover and hawthorn berry, work independently as an overall tonic for the body. Others, such as lavender and peppermint, work together to create a more pronounced healing effect. This 'working together' is called synergism and it is the basis of herbal medicine.

The key to good herbal medicine is in the blending of herbs to achieve a beneficial effect on individual symptoms. Take, for example, a common cold. In treating this I would blend four herbs to make a tea: elderflower, to stimulate perspiration and lower body temperature; garlic, which acts as an antibacterial; ginger, to dispel mucus and carry the other herbs throughout the body; and peppermint, whose essential oil clears the breathing passages. I often add honey, which lends antiseptic properties and adds flavour.

As well as treating ailments, herbal tea's other most important function is to maintain a sense of well-being. A body needs continual maintenance to keep it running smoothly. Herbal teas play a role in maintaining equilibrium. Along with a healthy diet, herbal teas help to keep the internal organs in top condition and improve the quality of life.

Herbal teas, used regularly and astutely, can prevent imbalances. For example, drinking about three cups of peppermint tea a day, particularly after meals, aids digestion and tunes the entire system. Peppermint tea can be used as a soothing and refreshing after-dinner drink following a heavy fatty meal, as it cuts through fats and renders them more digestible. Similarly, a cup of peppermint tea following a cup of coffee will ensure that the coffee (and the milk in a cappuccino) does not stress the system. Apres tea contains aniseed and fennel, which further aid the digestion of foods. Chamomile tea taken before bed calms, soothes and helps prevent insomnia. Two cups of Petal tea a day will maintain healthy, glowing skin. For sugar cravings, try Triple E tea. The liquorice root in this tea gives a sweet taste and helps to dispel the need for a sugar hit. Berry tea, a favourite of older people, helps to promote energy and vitality and has a rich flavour that is very satisfying.

Following is a discussion of the most common

ailments I see which can be treated very effectively with herbal teas. I have also included some case studies, which illustrate the therapeutic effects of herbal tea more clearly. You might find you have something in common with some of the people and the situations depicted in the case studies.

Allergies and respiratory problems

Patients often complain of allergic reactions to food or airborne irritants and report problems such as skin rashes, bronchial coughs, asthma, sinus blockage and upset stomach or bowels, such as irritable bowel. In some cases, food poisoning can be seen as an extreme allergy. Repeated respiratory viruses are an allied problem. Colds, coughs, flu, shortness of breath and bronchitis are complaints that I commonly treat with herbal teas. Patients who are susceptible to constant respiratory problems may, like allergy sufferers, suffer a hereditary weakness.

Australia is home to a host of unusual plants with potent pollens that can aggravate existing allergies or respiratory ailments such as asthma. Keeping the upper respiratory tract healthy can prevent infections in the lower respiratory tract, which may be harder to shift. Summer Delight tea, with its combination of peppermint, lemon thyme, spearmint and other herbs, can give great relief to sufferers of allergic or other respiratory conditions.

Case studies

A man in his fifties consulted me about his allergic reaction to strong odours, all perfumes and a general sensitivity to chemicals and synthetics in pollutants, washing soaps and detergents. He led a very busy lifestyle that involved eating out frequently. I prescribed two pots (a pot of tea being approximately four cups) of Summer Delight tea a day, to be taken after all meals, including after dining out at restaurants.

He took to the tea with great enthusiasm and even arranged for his own special stock to be kept at his favourite restaurants. He believed the tea had a calming effect on his whole constitution and found that it was a naturally pleasing scent to him. He even insisted that it appeared to increase his libido!

Another patient came to me complaining of strong allergic reactions during spring and autumn. He sneezed constantly, suffered from a runny nose and blocked sinuses, swollen red eyes and occasionally itchy skin. At first I prescribed a tea called 'eyebright' (also known as euphrasia) to be taken five to six times a day. I also asked him to bathe his eyes each morning with this infusion. I then recommended that he drink peppermint tea to relieve sinus congestion, and that he inhale the vapour of this tea to clear his upper respiratory tract.

His allergic reactions dropped markedly after ten days. On the next visit I asked him to mix the two teas together and add chamomile, to alleviate his skin reactions. After three weeks of taking these teas, he returned to me and reported that he felt much more clear-headed. The irritation of his eyes and skin had disappeared and sneezing bouts were now very rare.

Allergies can be seen as an imbalance of our internal and external environments. A patient who is run-down or otherwise unwell may respond adversely to changes in the weather or display a particular sensitivity to a chemical or pollutant. A hereditary predisposition makes the body particularly sensitive to certain conditions.

Teas can be used to desensitise the body. Put another way, tea allows the body to summon and strengthen its resources against the hostile elements to which it is susceptible. This means that while allergies may linger, their symptoms are reduced with proper treatment.

Respiratory problems are commonly passed around within family groups and I often treat entire families, especially at the beginning of the cold and flu season. Teas are an excellent preparation, as their gentle but effective action can be enjoyed by the young and old alike. The following infusion is suitable for everyone, including children over eight years old, and will improve the symptoms of colds, flu, laryngitis, bronchitis and asthma.

Other herbs that I use in a tea to expel the mucus of bronchial complaints are elecampane, spearmint, thyme and hot herbs such as ginger and cayenne.

A TEA FOR THE RELIEF OF RESPIRATORY PROBLEMS

Mix two teaspoons of liquorice root, two teaspoons of elderflower, two cloves of fresh garlic (crushed), one teaspoon of freshly chopped ginger, one teaspoon of peppermint and three teaspoons of honey. Place these ingredients in a pot and add four to five cups of water. Simmer on the stove for fifteen minutes; strain and drink regularly.

Digestion

With all the rigours of a stressful lifestyle, it is often the digestive system that starts to show the strain. Acid stomach, heartburn, hiatus hernia, peptic ulcer and halitosis (bad breath) are all problems associated with bad digestion. Constipation, diarrhoea, irritable bowel (which is often a combination of the two preceding symptoms), haemorrhoids, and even diverticulitis (inflamed pockets in the bowel wall) are problems that I commonly treat.

Lifestyle factors play a vital role in the regulation of digestion. Diet regulation is crucial for healthy bowel movement and for avoiding the simple but uncomfortable sensation of indigestion. Apart from a poorly functioning bowel and colon, the liver and pancreas are often under siege from unhealthy elements. The liver detoxifies and filters the blood, and if it is overloaded with fats and alcohol it will not perform well. A diet high in refined sugar will put stress on the pancreas, which controls the sugar levels in the blood.

If the liver, gall bladder and/or pancreas become sluggish, certain symptoms arise.

An inefficient liver or gall bladder can lead to fatigue, nausea, high cholesterol levels, bloating and the whites of the eyes becoming grey or veiny; a weak pancreas can result in highs and lows of energy, and, in extreme cases, diabetes.

Case study

A man came to see me complaining of stress and fatigue and an unbearable itch all over his body. After checking his iris and discussing his lifestyle and medical history, I came to the conclusion that this was a person who had little or no time for his health. His eating habits were irregular, as were his bowel motions. His digestive system was toxic from eating the wrong food and his whole system was suffering. His stressful job exacerbated the problem.

He admitted that it was his wife's idea to consult me and that he had done so only to keep the peace. I knew then that recommending radical changes to his diet and lifestyle would not work. Here was a very resistant patient who had to be treated through subtle but effective adjustments to his bad habits.

The only dietary change I recommended was that he eat some cereal every morning and that he have a regular salad and protein sandwich at lunchtime. However, in addition I asked him to drink six cups of Triple E tea a day. This tea is rich in liquorice root, which would regularise his bowel motions. Liquorice root also mimics a cortico-steroid action, which would have an anti-inflammatory effect on his itch. After three weeks, his feeling of wellbeing had returned and his energy levels had increased by at least fifty per cent.

I kept him to this program for three months and introduced other herbal teas, but he was never as keen on any other flavour. To this day he drinks Triple E tea as a preventive beverage and because he enjoys the flavour.

Teas can be tailored to reduce the effects of a bad diet and irregular eating habits. Often, the simple addition of more fluid to the diet through the drinking of a few cups of tea a day will work wonders and aid digestive function generally. I sometimes find that patients are unwilling or unable to change their diet; however, they can always add tea to their routine. Tea taken in this way can counteract the other elements, which may be harmful, although ideally tea should be a complement to a healthy lifestyle.

There are certain teas that should always be kept in store and taken regularly to promote efficient digestion. Peppermint tea at the end of a meal high in fats and alcohol will allow the body to restore equilibrium as peppermint helps the body metabolise fat. Any bitter herbal tea, such as dandelion tea, is good for the liver. Lemon juice in hot water, which I classify as a herbal drink, is a great start to the day for those who are prone to bad digestion. Fluctuations in energy levels due to poor sugar metabolism can be aided by drinking liquorice tea because its slightly sweet flavour assuages the craving for sugar that often plagues those with a poorly functioning pancreas. Liquorice also assists in regulating bowel motions. Meadowsweet tea counteracts heartburn and slippery elm tea assists irritable bowel by regulating and healing inflammation.

Fatigue and circulatory problems

Many, many patients who come to see me start their session by saying 'I feel tired and run-down, and I don't have any energy'. Lifestyle factors play an enormous part in determining an individual's vitality and sense of wellbeing. Poor eating habits, lack of fluid and a sedentary job often lead to underactive digestion and iron deficiency, resulting in fatigue and lack of energy. Stress is another factor that influences vitality. In addition, many people simply do not get enough sleep or even time to rest and recuperate quietly.

Circulatory problems can also result from these same lifestyle problems. A sluggish blood flow can lead to fatigue, varicose veins and heart conditions. Poor diet and inadequate fluid intake are, once again, the culprits here. Bad circulation will also affect the brain and memory. It is interesting to note that scans of the brains of sufferers of Alzheimer's disease show pronounced dehydration.

Case studies

A mother of three children under six came to see me 'frazzled, tired and at the end of her tether', as she put it. I was concerned that she may be low in iron, so I sent her to her doctor for a blood test, which proved that her iron levels were indeed very low. She was reluctant to take iron tablets because she already suffered from constipation. On examining her diet more carefully, I discovered that she drank up to ten cups of black tea a day. The tannin in black tea can play havoc with iron absorption, so I asked her to reduce her tea intake to two cups per day, and to take Triple E tea as often as she could. I prescribed Triple

E because it would help to re-energise her exhausted adrenal glands as well as give her energy. The tea would also help her overcome the constipation associated with taking iron tablets.

She reported a major improvement within a month. She told me that she made up a large glass plunger of tea every morning and drank it hot and cold throughout the day, adding water to the used herbs when needed. She was happy to be experiencing real, refreshing sleep, and she was a lot less irritable with her children. Another welcome by-product of her new tea-drinking ritual was that she lost a few extra kilograms, as the tea helped her digestion and her bowels.

Many men complain of weight, circulatory and energy problems. Often they are all connected. One male patient, still a young man in his mid-thirties, consulted me about his weight and his lack of energy. He led an extremely hectic life and was not receptive to drastic changes in his diet or lifestyle. He said that he really did not have time for exercise.

Because of his resistance, I started gently. I asked him to drink two glasses of warm boiled water or lemongrass and buchu (excellent for flushing out the kidneys) tea every morning, sweetened with honey or flavoured with lemon, if he wished. I asked him to repeat this every three hours for ten days. I allowed him two alcoholic drinks, one coffee and one black tea per day.

In ten days his improvement was marked. He lost two kilograms and passed a number of kidney stones. He felt much better and his confidence improved. He was then a lot more receptive to other changes in his diet, which I introduced slowly.

To restore energy and vitality, Berry tea – which contains hawthorn berry – is helpful. Chamomile tea is always excellent for winding down the system and encouraging sleep. Chamomile tea's calming effect can be useful to simply lower stress levels during the day and maintain equilibrium. For long-term fatigue, ginseng tea mixed with ginger is excellent. Liquorice tea will help exhausted adrenal glands, while bitter herbal teas, such as dandelion, will stimulate the appetite, often a problem associated with exhaustion.

Many young people ask me to provide them with a herbal remedy for the excesses of a big night out. The effects of profuse perspiration and fatigue from lack of sleep can be minimised by drinking a special tea throughout the night. Made from liquorice, ginseng and peppermint, this tea is refreshing and has a pleasant, invigorating taste. Guarana can be added, as well as honey (for energy) and a teaspoon of magnesium. Magnesium assists in restoring electrolyte balance, which can be disturbed by perspiration. It also helps to break down lactic acid build-up from vigorous dancing!

Dandelion and lemongrass tea will speed up recovery the next day. Dandelion root is a marvellous liver tonic, and lemongrass flushes out toxins. Slippery elm tea will soothe heartburn associated with drinking too much alcohol.

Hormonal imbalances

Tension associated with premenstrual syndrome (PMS), fluid retention, menopause, irregular menstrual periods and hormonal skin break-outs are very common female ailments that can be treated with a range of teas. *Agnus castus* or 'chaste tree' tea is very effective in soothing the symptoms of PMS. Chamomile and Petal teas will alleviate problems of mood swings and skin break-outs.

Case studies

A menopausal woman came to see me complaining of depression, loss of vitality, lack of motivation, insomnia and hot flushes. For most of her life she had been a high achiever, and she was most distressed by her problems. She was not on any hormone replacement therapy because of a family history of breast cancer.

As this patient found it difficult to swallow tablets and disliked taking medication of any kind,

I treated her with sage tea. While this tea can have an unpleasant taste, it is marvellous in treating menopausal symptoms. It can be sweetened with honey or another tea can be added to improve the flavour. In this case, I added a little lemongrass tea with dandelion leaves to dispel the fluid retention around her ankles and thighs.

My patient returned after six weeks reporting regained confidence and vitality, diminished hot flushes and much improved sleep.

Another woman came to see me about her moodiness, aggression and skin break-outs. She could not tell me exactly when these bouts seemed to be at their worst, so I gave her a diary to fill out and asked her to return in a month. Sure enough, her symptoms started to appear strongly two weeks before her period, and I diagnosed hormonal imbalance as the problem.

From day ten of her cycle (which is ten days

after her period began, or about eighteen days before the next was due), I asked her to drink three cups of chamomile tea and three cups of Petal tea a day. The red clover in Petal tea helps to cleanse the lymphatic system thereby clearing the skin as well as correcting slight hormonal imbalances. Chamomile is also present in Petal tea, but this patient needed extra chamomile to calm her aggression and moodiness. Chamomile also helps calm allergic, heated skin conditions.

The only supplement I prescribed was evening primrose oil: 2000 milligrams in the morning and 2000 milligrams in the evening (these capsules must contain ten per cent gamma-linolenic acid).

The following month her diary read quite differently. Her skin broke out slightly only one day before her period and returned to normal very quickly. The moodiness and irritability she had earlier reported did not reappear. She noted some sugar cravings about five days before her period was due, and I advised her to drink sweet teas such as liquorice root or Berry tea, as well as eating small protein snacks every three hours.

Women needn't suffer unnecessarily with hormone-related ailments when herbal teas can effectively alleviate many of the symptoms. Certain teas can be very helpful in pregnancy and to prepare a woman's body for labour. Three cups a day of red raspberry leaf tea, traditionally known to help strengthen the womb for labour, can be safely used in the last six to eight weeks of pregnancy. In cases of post-partum depression, I advise drinking two cups of chaste tree tea a day to help the hormones return to their normal balance. However, it is important to see a herbalist before taking any herbal tea while pregnant.

Joint and muscular pain

Painful joints and muscles can be treated effectively with herbs. Many patients consult me with problems associated with joint and ligament deterioration. They often complain of muscular aches and pains, rheumatism and arthritis.

Case study

An elderly man was brought to me by his daughter. He was suffering from swollen sore joints, which he described as arthritis, and very cold feet that cramped at night. His digestion was poor so he was reluctant to take tablets. Fortunately he loved the taste of ginger, so I prescribed fresh ginger tea, made by cutting up two teaspoons of fresh ginger, adding it to two cups of boiling water, and either letting it stand for twenty minutes or boiling it for ten minutes. I advised him to drink at least four cups of this tea a day. For his feet I prescribed a chamomile foot bath (see page 69) every night.

These remedies were gentle but very effective, and after around four months he gained much symptomatic relief from following this regimen.

Lactic acid build-up is often responsible for the ache felt in muscles. The best way of moving the lactic acid build-up is to increase fluid intake. Muscles and joints may ache after too much exercise, but they will also lock up under stress and the passive pressures of a sedentary lifestyle.

Older people are often subject to aches and pains in joints and muscles, and need to increase their fluid intake. They often make the mistake of drinking too much black tea, which contains tannin. Tannin interferes with nutrient absorption. Many herbal teas do not contain tannin and have therapeutic properties that can assist in the removal of toxins. At the same time, herbal teas also treat the affliction for which they are prescribed.

In general, nettle tea is very effective in treating rheumatism and arthritis, although burdock and yellow dock teas also have been used traditionally to address joint pain. Ginger, with the addition of a pinch of cayenne pepper for extra effect, warms the body and stimulates circulation. Meadowsweet tea contains traces of salicylate, which can be useful in controlling acid and pain in the joints. Liquorice, with its anti-inflammatory effect, is another useful herb.

Skin, hair and nail problems

Itchy skin rashes, including eczema and psoriasis; dull and brittle hair and nails; acne; and fine white pimples under the skin are problems that often respond well to treatment with herbal teas.

These symptoms can be associated with a number of problems, and may even be part of a hereditary pattern. An overload of sugar, fatty or acidic foods such as citrus or small seed fruit, poor digestion affecting mineral uptake, and stress can also play a part. I see more of these problems in female patients, because hormonal fluctuations are often a major factor. They can also be associated with allergic reactions. Many more patients complain about these symptoms in winter, because some types of skin suffer from irritation when clothed constantly and when heavier, starchy foods are eaten.

Case study

A young woman came to see me complaining of small whitehead pimples that had broken out on her face, particularly on her forehead, nose and chin. Her skin also had red patches in places. She told me that she never drank water, but did consume large quantities of sweet fizzy drinks, which are loaded with sugar, preservatives and artificial colouring.

I prescribed Petal tea, because of its high content of red clover which acts as a lymphatic cleanser. Chamomile and lavender, also present in the tea, have a calming effect on the skin. It was a big change for her to drink water, let alone herbal tea. Luckily, she enjoyed the taste of the tea, so drinking the required amount was not difficult.

After six weeks, her skin looked ninety per cent better. The quality of her skin changed, with her face regaining a glowing, refreshed look. She also commented that her circulation seemed to have improved due to the greater fluid content she was ingesting. Her hair and nails had also strengthened and were not breaking as easily. I advised her to continue to take Petal tea as prescribed and to add one to two cups of horsetail tea per day to further strengthen her hair and nails.

The intake of fluid that is the simple result of drinking herbal tea is in itself a great tonic for the skin. Teas to store in the cupboard to keep skin in prime condition are Petal, red clover and peppermint teas. Horsetail strengthens hair and nails. Chamomile is especially good for allergic skin reactions to pollens in spring and autumn.

Dandelion helps to remove poisons from the liver which may be showing in the skin. Burdock and yellow dock teas are classed as blood purifiers and often assist with stubborn cases of acne. Garlic, with its high sulphur content, helps to purify blood and clear the complexion.

Stress and anxiety

Panic and anxiety attacks, insomnia, depression and difficulty coping all signal overloaded stress levels and anxiety. As with problems related to energy levels, lifestyle factors are critical. Often these patients need advice in crisis management. Sometimes the prescription of antidepressants is indicated. Treatment with tea can be very effective in controlling some of the symptoms of anxiety.

Case studies

The managing director of a very large company consulted me because he was experiencing symptoms of stress. However, even though he knew he was run-down, he didn't really want to change his dietary habits. My approach was simply to increase his fluid intake by recommending he drink at least six to eight cups of fluid a day, preferably in the form of herbal teas.

When he returned six weeks later, he told me he couldn't believe how much better he felt. He had taken to drinking chamomile tea all day, which he said was his favourite. I asked him if he felt at all sleepy after drinking such large quantities of chamomile tea, but he said it simply made him feel more relaxed and healthy. He laughingly told me that the only side effect was during the first week, when he almost called boardroom meetings in the bathroom due to the tea's 'flushing' effect! I also observed that the psoriasis on his hands had improved dramatically.

Teenage girls often come to me citing problems with anxiety and eating disorders. An eighteen-year-old girl suffering from anorexia and panic attacks was brought to me by her very concerned mother. I knew that the psychological problems associated with anorexic behaviour would make it difficult for me to impose a new eating regime, so I chose to treat the young girl with tea.

I made a tea blend from a number of herbal teas: chamomile to relax her and soothe the stomach lining; lemon verbena to alleviate the anxiety and lend a pleasant taste; a pinch of liquorice to stimulate her tastebuds and help relieve the constipation that often goes with eating disorders; and a touch of lemongrass and buchu tea to improve kidney function. Lastly, I also added some peppermint to stimulate the appetite. I asked her to make a glass plunger (approximately eight glasses) every morning and drink it throughout the day hot or at room temperature.

The tea virtually eliminated her panic attacks and soothed her digestive tract. It enabled the bowel to move regularly and had a slight diuretic effect. The tea could not help cure her anorexia, but it did help relieve some of its distressing symptoms.

Certain teas can have powerful calming effects and should be kept on hand for the general treatment of stress and anxiety. Chamomile and vervain teas are reliable remedies. Berry tea is also excellent for these conditions. Passionflower tea addresses the problem of insomnia; ginseng tea helps lift depression. Rosemary tea with basil improves mood and when mixed with peppermint works well as a treatment for minor depression. Traditionally, the fresh leaf of the feverfew herb was chewed to dispel migraines. Feverfew tea alleviates the headaches that are often associated with stress and anxiety.

4

essential

herbs

M any people ask me what are my favourite herbs for herbal teas. Following is a brief exploration of these herbs and why they are so useful in teas.

Chamomile

One of the safest and most widely used herbs, chamomile is renowned for being a powerful relaxant suitable for both internal and external use. It is especially effective when used to treat problems of the digestive tract or to soothe rashes and allergic skin conditions. It is also excellent as a treatment for anxiety and stress, and has long been known to help insomnia.

Chamomile has a celebrated history as a calmative. Favoured by the Greeks and Romans and referred to frequently in many ancient medical texts, we now know chamomile contains natural oils that hold the key to its effectiveness. One of these oils, chamazulene, has strong anti-inflammatory properties and is a natural sedative. Chamomile also contains another therapeutic substance called dicyclic ether, a natural anti-spasmodic. This enables chamomile to relieve uncomfortable spasms in the intestine due to poor digestion and alleviate nausea, vomiting and diarrhoea. It also works well for women who suffer painful menstrual periods.

The chamomile plant can grow to over sixty centimetres in height, but it is the fragrant yellow flowers that are essential in the production of tea. The addition of boiling water releases the tea's essential oil and distinctive aroma. Therefore the most effective way to experience the benefits of chamomile is to use it as a tea. Two or three cups of chamomile tea taken throughout the day will relieve digestive problems, allergic reactions and anxiety. A strong cup (two teaspoons to one cup of boiling water) of chamomile taken before bedtime will induce a sound sleep.

A CHAMOMILE TEA BATH

For a foot or hand bath, add two tablespoons of chamomile tea to two cups of boiling water. Let the tea infuse; strain and add to a basin filled with one litre of warm water. Soak feet or hands for ten to fifteen minutes.

For a full body bath, fill a small muslin bag with one to two tablespoons of chamomile tea. Tie the bag and float it in a warm bath where it will continue to infuse for the length of your bath. If you haven't a muslin bag handy, then make a pot of chamomile tea and add it to the bath. Relax by drinking a cup or two of the tea as you soak.

Chamomile is also used to treat peripheral circulatory problems. Chamomile tea will help to ease a headache or when added to a foot bath will relieve tired or swollen feet. This makes it useful for elderly patients who suffer from problems associated with restricted circulation. Bathing in water infused with chamomile soothes chilblains, varicose veins and the aches associated with poor circulation. With its anti-inflammatory properties, chamomile in a tea bath will soothe arthritic joints and allergic skin rashes.

Tired and itchy eyes benefit from the application of damp chamomile teabags or cotton wool balls impregnated with tea to closed eyelids. Place the teabags or cotton balls over the eyelids and rest for ten minutes to feel the benefits.

Because it is gentle as well as powerful, chamomile is excellent for children. Used to wash delicate young skin, cooled chamomile tea helps relieve the pain of nappy rash or other skin irritations and allergies. When tea is added to milk or drunk in a weak infusion (add some honey to make it more palatable, if necessary), it relieves sleeplessness and irritability due to teething. It can also be used to simply wind down a restless or excited child.

A CHAMOMILE HAIR RINSE

People with blond hair – true blonds and assisted blonds equally – will be pleased to know that chamomile can be used as a beauty aid. Make up a cup of chamomile tea using one tablespoon of tea to one cup of boiling water. Let it cool, and rinse the strained tea through your hair after washing. Do not rinse it out. The chamomile rinse gives an added lustre to your locks.

Drinking chamomile tea after a heavy or rich meal will settle the stomach and allow for a restful sleep. My Apres tea contains a strong dose of chamomile. Designed to be taken after meals, Apres can be used any time for upset digestion, and is suitable for both adults and children. Containing chamomile, fennel (to soothe the pancreas), peppermint (for the gall bladder) and aniseed (to relax the stomach muscles), the recipe was adapted from a very old herbal remedy for disturbed digestion. I have also prescribed Apres tea to relieve problems such as premenstrual syndrome, menopause-related insomnia, or general nervousness due to work pressure or exams.

Dandelion

Tea made from the roots and leaves of dandelions has been used traditionally throughout the East to treat complaints of the liver. Today, researchers are trying to determine why it is so effective and are searching for a western scientific explanation for something herbalists have known about for many hundreds of years.

We know that dandelion tea works wonders on a sluggish liver (the primary filtering organ of the body), gall bladder (which produces bile to assist the digestion of fatty foods) and spleen (an organ producing new red blood cells), and that it encourages bowel action and reduces fluid retention. Drinking dandelion tea is one of the most effective ways to detoxify your body, because it stimulates digestive enzymes and bile to allow the easier metabolism of fatty foods.

It is essential to use the right sort of herbs for this tea, because one of the properties of the plant is to absorb metal pollutants from the atmosphere. For this reason, organically grown dandelion is essential. The root is the most potent part of the plant and can be used in piece or powder form. It can be a little bitter, but the taste improves to a refreshing tartness when mixed with honey and even milk. When lemongrass is added to dandelion tea, it has a tonic effect on sluggish kidneys.

Dandelion tea is excellent for ridding the body of excess fluid. As the tea leaves contain high amounts of potassium, the body is not depleted of this important mineral through the diuretic effect of the tea.

Ginger

Ginger has a wide range of uses and is one of the most important herbs in a herbalist's repertoire. It is one of the finest herbs used to stimulate circulation, lift sagging moods and improve vitality.

The Chinese hold ginger in high esteem and refer to it as a 'heating' herb that increases vitality, a concept associated with warmth. I have found that it has a marked effect on patients who spend a lot of time in the water or the snow and come to me complaining of cold hands and feet. I recommend that they take ginger tea both before and after a session in the water or on the slopes, and their condition always improves. Warming and stimulating, the effect of ginger tea is heightened with a pinch of cayenne pepper. It is also delicious mixed with cinnamon and cloves, and children may enjoy it taken this way with a spoonful of honey.

It is therefore a wonderful tea to be used in the treatment of arthritis, cold hands and feet, and nausea, and is excellent at eliminating mucus in bronchial conditions. I often use ginger in the treatment of older patients, as it is excellent in the treatment of joint and circulatory problems.

Ginger tea is easily prepared by adding half to one teaspoon of grated ginger root to one cup of boiling water twice a day. Dried ginger tea is often a little bit stronger, so it is recommended that you use less of it. Ginger can also be added safely to any other tea. A good example is a mixture of peppermint and ginger. While the peppermint works independently to clear mucus, the ginger works synergistically to carry the effect throughout the body.

A COMPRESS FOR PAINFUL MENSTRUAL PERIODS

Add two teaspoons of grated ginger root to two cups of water. Simmer for fifteen to twenty minutes. Soak a clean piece of lint or towelling in the mixture, wring out excess liquid and apply to the affected area. Leave for ten to fifteen minutes, then repeat.

Sipping hot ginger tea during a painful menstrual period can work wonders. A hot pack of ginger applied directly to the abdomen is a traditional and effective way to relieve stomach cramps, especially in young teenage girls.

Ginseng

Ginseng has the ability to maintain and assist vitality in myriad ways. It can help patients recover from prolonged stress, a long illness, or shock and trauma. Siberian and Korean ginseng are effective used in a tea, although for a stronger therapeutic effect ginseng is best used in tablet or tincture form. Tea can be made from the dried roots, which can be cut or broken and steeped for ten or fifteen minutes in boiling water. Because of its bitter taste, it can be mixed with another tea or honey to taste.

Siberian ginseng seems to work especially well when patients have to contend with adverse working or environmental conditions. It improves stamina and increases mental and physical output. Russian athletes have used this herb to strengthen their capacity for endurance and concentration. It appears to inhibit the side effects of chemotherapy and surgery, and aids the healing process. It also assists libido and has even been shown in some cases to increase sperm count when ingested in therapeutic doses over a period of time.

Korean ginseng improves the body's ability to deal with stress. Improvements in concentration, stamina and stress resistance are often reported when taking Korean ginseng.

While studies have recorded a general absence of side effects, it is advisable to use Siberian and Korean ginseng in consultation with a herbalist because of their strength as stimulants. I recommend taking ginseng for three to four months during prolonged stress, then to take a break for six to eight weeks.

Hawthorn

This herb is a proven vascular tonic and an extraordinary antioxidant, and promotes the wellbeing of the entire cardiovascular system. It is especially helpful at counter-acting the ageing process because it strengthens vascular fragility, reduces atherosclerosis (cholesterol build-up in arteries) and varicose veins, and soothes the discomfort of menopause. It improves the flow of blood through the coronary arteries and increases general vitality.

Patients with high or low blood pressure benefit from drinking hawthorn tea. It works effectively on patients who suffer from panic attacks or nervous insomnia because it acts as a sedative and assists in regulating hypertension.

Many of my older patients do very well on Berry tea, which has a large component of hawthorn. Another ingredient in this tea is elderberry. The elder tree is sacred to gypsies because it is said to protect other herbs and because it is believed to be the tree from which Christ's cross was made. Juniper, another component of Berry tea, has delicious, strong flavours and a slight diuretic effect.

Lemongrass

Traditionally, lemongrass was a tonic for the skin and eyes. This straw-like plant or grass has long been used for flavour in Thai cooking. Because of its pleasant taste, lemongrass is a good tea to use in combination with other teas that may lack flavour or are unpleasant to taste. It is a refreshing tea for tropical climates and can be drunk hot or cold.

Lemongrass has a number of important properties. Its diuretic effect aids the kidneys, its volatile lemon oil cuts through fats related to heavy meals, and its sedative effect calms the nervous system.

Lemongrass also has antifungal properties. I often use it for patients who suffer from candidiasis (the infection caused by the fungus *Candida albicans*) and mild skin irritations. There has been some debate

A NOTE ON LAVENDER IN TEA

As a herb, lavender has exceptional calming properties, but it needs to be carefully used when brewing tea. Used on its own, it can be overwhelming enough to cause nausea – even the very diluted mix of half a teaspoon to one cup of boiling water is too much for some people. Because the essential oil in this herb is very strong, lavender is best used in combination with other teas. My Petal tea blends lavender with chamomile, red clover and rose petals to create a relaxing, anti-stress brew. I also recommend adding a pinch of lavender to chamomile tea to enhance the sedative effect.

Lavender oil is marvellous when used in a bath to encourage muscle relaxation. If you do not have lavender oil handy, then make a tea by adding one teaspoon of lavender to two to three cups of boiling water. When cooled, simply add the tea to your bath (do not drink the brew).

about whether herbal teas should be used at all in the treatment of candidiasis, as some practitioners believe that all tea is fermented and that fermentation can encourage candidiasis. However, it is important to point out that only black tea is fermented; herbal tea is not (see chapter 2).

Liquorice

Used for centuries as a treatment for coughs and other bronchial complaints such as influenza and asthma, recent research shows that this herb also helps adrenal glands to recover after long periods of stress. Liquorice contains glycosides, which are fifty times sweeter than sugar. This makes the taste of liquorice tea appealing, especially for those patients with a sweet tooth. (Beware of commercial confectionery called liquorice – most of it is sweetened with high quantities of sugar and flavoured with aniseed oil. These sweets hold little therapeutic benefit.)

Liquorice tea is an excellent treatment for stomach cramps, indigestion caused by too much stomach acid, and ulcers of both the stomach and the mouth, because it also contains strong anti-inflammatory properties. Another key ingredient in liquorice root has an effect similar to synthetic cortisone, which explains its effectiveness in treating exhaustion of the adrenal glands. (In western medicine, cortisone is often prescribed for adrenal cortex malfunction.) What this means is that liquorice is excellent in counteracting exhaustion due to physical exertion or prolonged illness. This ingredient also makes liquorice tea useful as a wash for psoriasis and eczema, conditions that are often treated with cortisone creams.

Triple E tea is so named to indicate that it offers a triple dose of energy. It contains liquorice, peppermint and aniseed – herbs that work synergistically to soothe, calm and purify the colon as well as stimulate mood and tastebuds. It restores energy in stressful conditions.

Nettle

In ancient times, the stinging nettle was steamed and eaten as a vegetable (it is high in vitamins A and C). Tea made with nettles has been used over the ages to treat a range of problems. It has been used to assist milk production in women and animals, and by herbalists to treat adult-onset diabetes, although we are still not sure exactly why it works in this way. Similarly, it seems to prevent hair loss and has often been used in hair tonics.

Today, herbalists use nettle to treat a wide range of illnesses. Because of its high iron content and nutritional qualities, nettle tea is useful in the treatment of anaemia and fatigue. Taken regularly, it soothes aches and pains in joints, muscles and ligaments associated with arthritis, rheumatism, gout and uric acid retention. A nettle tea foot bath dissipates gout and swelling. These foot baths were used regularly by English and French kings in the fifteenth and sixteenth centuries who indulged in rich foods and suffered uric acid build-up. A three-litre foot bath containing an infusion of tea (two heaped teaspoons nettle added to three cups boiling water, cooled) and a tablespoon of Epsom salts, will stimulate circulation and drain uric acid.

Nettle can be quite bland in taste, and works well when mixed with chamomile and peppermint or simply with a spoonful of honey.

Passionflower

This is the same plant that produces passionfruit, but herbalists use the leaves to make a tea that is exceptionally useful as a gentle sedative and relaxant. It is used to treat nervousness and anxiety, tachycardia (abnormally fast heartbeat), insomnia and nightmares. Mixed with chamomile, passionflower is especially safe for children.

Passionflower also alleviates the mood swings associated with premenstrual syndrome, mild depression, and the pain of neuralgia and shingles. Recent discoveries have found that passionflower encourages the uptake of tryptophan, which is an amino acid that assists deep sleep, as well as maintaining levels of serotonin, which is a hormone that is crucial in regulating mood swings and depression.

High doses of this herb should not be consumed during pregnancy.

Peppermint

Tea made from the leaves of the peppermint plant was highly prized in ancient Egypt and by the Hebrews. The plant is harvested just before the flowers open, and the leaves are carefully dried. Peppermint tea is the favourite drink of Moroccan Arabs, who always conclude their rich meals with copious quantities of this most refreshing of brews.

The peppermint plant is full of the natural oil methal (or menthol) which has antiseptic, calming, antispasmodic and mucus-inhibiting qualities. Peppermint is especially good for relaxing the gall bladder, which allows bile to flow more freely and thus assists digestion, especially for sufferers of acid stomach or dyspepsia. It 'cuts through' fatty foods and allows them to be digested more smoothly. Peppermint tea relaxes the muscles of the stomach and bowel and reduces flatulence.

Menthol acts as a mild anaesthetic to the mucous lining of the stomach wall, and so reduces nausea. For this reason, it is recommended for travel sickness and morning sickness in pregnancy. Menthol is also very soothing to mucus congestion in the nose and has long been used as an ingredient in inhalants. Drinking peppermint tea has the same effect. It also has an uplifting effect on mood without being a stimulant, and should be used to promote a sense of calm concentration. Peppermint tea is invigorating, while at the same time it reduces anxiety and tension.

One of the major attractions of peppermint tea is its delicious taste. It can be drunk hot or cold. Ice blocks for children made from peppermint tea and honey are an excellent alternative to the sugar- and chemical-laden commercial varieties. Cold peppermint tea invigorates the mind and body in enervating humidity or heat.

TEA AND RED WINE

Many people have likened Berry tea to a good glass of red wine. I call Berry tea my 'red wine' tea because, like red wine, it has a naturally high content of flavonoids, which are effective antioxidants. However, it can be safely drunk all night without the side effects of alcohol.

Red wine is one of the richest sources of flavonoids. It is thought that this is the reason for the French Paradox: while the French enjoy an opulent diet, they also have a relatively low incidence of coronary heart disease, possibly due to the red wine imbibed with the rich cheese and sauces. Replete with flavonoids, the red wine counteracts the unhealthy consumption of too much fat and dairy produce.

Raspberry

Used often to treat women, raspberry leaf tea (also known as red raspberry) is especially good for pregnancy and strengthening the uterus. It is used to alleviate the nausea of morning sickness, as well as to encourage lactation in nursing mothers. For women who experience heavy menstrual periods, raspberry can help to decrease menstrual flow without stopping it abruptly.

I always prescribe raspberry leaf tea two months before a pregnant woman's labour is due. I also recommend it to women who are prone to miscarriages – to be taken between the time of miscarriage and falling pregnant – as well as throughout the entire pregnancy.

In higher doses, raspberry can improve constipation, which many women complain of during pregnancy. I have often prescribed it – mixed with chamomile and peppermint – for children suffering from diarrhoea.

Red clover

For centuries, red clover has been used as a lymphatic 'drainer' or detoxifying herb for the lymphatic system. It is a marvellous skin cleanser because the health of the lymphatic system is a factor influencing the health of the skin. It is also used to treat breast congestion, and breast and ovarian cancers. Poultices of this herb, applied directly, were used traditionally to treat lumps or tumours of the breast.

Red clover is an extremely effective, yet mysterious, plant, and research presently being conducted is only just beginning to understand the scientific reasons for its beneficial effects, especially in relation to hormonal imbalances at menopause.

This plant is used in Petal tea for keeping the skin clear and fresh. The tea is gentle enough for children to ingest.

Sage

An acquired taste, sage tea is an essential tonic for women who suffer from the mood swings and night sweats of menopause. As with red clover, the exact reasons behind the therapeutic effects of sage are not fully understood, but herbalists know that sage tea can reduce excessive sweating and lift the depression associated with menopause. Indeed, taken regularly, it can rescue women from the despair that often accompanies the 'change of life'.

Sage is an astringent and antiseptic herb. Up to thirty per cent of the volatile oil content in sage is thujone, a natural antiseptic. The astringent qualities of sage mean that it protects inflamed areas in the body. Sage is therefore an excellent mouthwash for patients who suffer from sore throats and inflamed mouth ulcers. It is also useful as a mouthwash for inflamed gums following dental work.

Mixing sage with lemongrass tea can improve the taste markedly. Lemongrass calms and soothes, so this herb works in tandem with sage to deliver true healing effects.

HERBAL HEALING – WITH FOOT BATHS

Traditionally herbal tea foot baths and hand baths have been effective in treating ailments such as arthritis, headaches and skin conditions of the hands and feet, although the reasons for this are not clear. They are a particularly useful alternative to drinking unpleasant-tasting teas.

Slippery elm

Slippery elm is most often found in powdered form and comes from the bark of the *Ulmus fulva* tree, which is a native of North America. A marvellous soothing herb, it works very well in the treatment of internal and external inflammations of mucous membranes. Internally, this includes peptic ulcers, acid stomach, irritable bowel, diverticulitis, diarrhoea, dysentery and sore throats. Externally, it works well on burns, ulcers and wounds.

Slippery elm is also a mucilaginous herb. This means that when water is added, the powder becomes sticky and thick. This substance then acts as a poultice for the inflamed area, soothing it and preventing irritating substances from being absorbed. Therefore, it should be drunk *before* eating to line the painful area.

This herb is safe for use by children, and can even be sprinkled on cereal. For those who dislike the taste, slippery elm can be mixed with a little honey or sweetened yoghurt. A teaspoon in just over half a litre of boiled milk is excellent for weaning babies, which then prevents bowel complications. Slippery elm is useful for sore throats, and when taken before alcohol will line the stomach and slow down the absorption of the alcohol. It is also an excellent ingredient in a hangover cure or after eating rich food, as it alleviates acid stomach symptoms.

Thyme

The variety of thyme most often used to make tea is lemon thyme. The volatile oil in thyme works to suppress coughing, so thyme tea is used as a treatment for severe coughs, asthma and bronchitis. Its antiseptic and antibacterial properties help to modify intestinal flora, making it a useful herb for the treatment of digestive disorders. Thyme tea also improves the appetite.

Summer Delight tea uses lemon thyme to improve the general taste. Also, the strong antiseptic properties of lemon thyme work with spearmint and peppermint to invigorate the lungs and sinuses and add clarity to the mind.

Vervain

Revered by the druids as one of the seven sacred plants, vervain was traditionally named Holy Wort or Herb of Grace. It was used in Celtic magic and also by the

Romans, who dedicated the herb to Venus and included it in love potions.

Used widely in Europe and especially France as a sedative and calming tea, vervain is often avoided because many people find its bland taste unappealing. (To liven up the taste, I recommend mixing vervain tea with flavoursome and aromatic chamomile tea, which has similar properties.) However, the effectiveness of vervain as an anti-stress and restorative tea is undisputed, and it has been used for centuries to treat headaches and anxiety.

Vervain is especially useful as a restorative treatment after periods of long illness and chronic fatigue. It acts as a mood elevator, which makes this tea very useful as a treatment for mental and nervous exhaustion from overwork, or for bouts of depression. Interestingly, vervain was historically used to treat asthma and mild epilepsy.

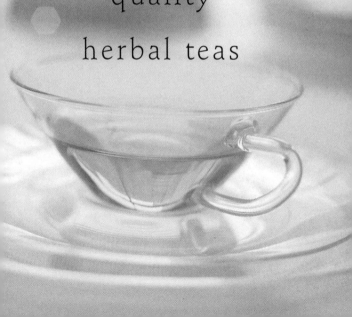

5

choosing

quality

herbal teas

Y ou have decided to drink herbal tea – but what is a *quality* herbal tea and how can you identify it? Before I can give you any helpful suggestions, you need to answer this fundamental question: do you want to drink herbal tea purely to experience a different taste sensation or are you hoping to achieve true health-giving benefits?

Teabags or loose-leaf tea?

As I explained earlier, only a small amount of tea can fit into a teabag. The actual amount, which is under two grams, is not sufficient to affect positive changes to your health and is therefore not considered a therapeutic substance. In addition, the herbs must be crushed or powdered to fit into the bag, a process that strips the herbs of their therapeutic essential oils. While there may remain traces of active ingredients in the tea, a herbal teabag is not the tea of choice if you are looking for the healing effects of herbal tea.

Teabags are great if you are simply after variety of flavour – and there is certainly plenty of variety! A range of herbal and fruit-flavoured teabags is readily available from supermarkets, and the range continues to expand. When choosing herbal teabags, be guided by your individual tastes. Some companies sell packs of assorted teabags so you can try a number of different flavours. Experiment with different brands and, to the best of your knowledge, choose a reputable company that is environmentally friendly.

If you are looking for more than just taste and are seeking the kinds of health-giving benefits that I've discussed in this book, you must choose high-quality, *loose-leaf* herbal teas. Loose-leaf teas have not undergone the harsh processing required for the manufacture of teabags, and subsequently they retain their therapeutic properties and their flavour. And as we use three to five grams to make a herbal tea (and can reuse the leaves to make a second and third cup), the healing potential of the tea is increased.

SOURCING HIGH-QUALITY HERBS

A good herbalist will always source the highest-quality herbs available. This means that the number of active ingredients in a tea, as well as its aroma, colour, taste, texture and purity is of a superior standard, and therefore will deliver the greatest health-giving effects.

Fragrance, colour and taste

The most important indicators of quality are fragrance, colour and taste. Strong aromas indicate a high level of essential oils, while dense colour and full-bodied taste show that other active ingredients are present. These factors tell you much about the quality of the herbs and the standards of processing, regardless of whether they are organic, wildcrafted or cultivated teas. Of course, you will not always be able to ascertain whether a tea is fragrant, colourful or tasty until you have bought it. Experiment with different teas and different manufacturers until you have found a high-quality tea to give you the effect you desire.

Organic, wildcrafted and cultivated teas

Many herbs are sprayed heavily with pesticides, as insects love the sweet flavours and aromas that herbs produce. Pesticides and other chemical additives weaken the flavour and therapeutic value of the herbs, and might also be detrimental to our health.

Organically grown herbs have been cultivated without the use of pesticides and other chemicals.

Organic substances are used to enrich the soil, and insect-repellent plants are grown in and around the herbs. Wildcrafted herbs are similar: they are actually grown 'in the wild' without any controls whatsoever, and are therefore arguably of the highest quality. However, the demand for wildcrafted herbs has endangered some species. The absence of chemical interference with organic and wildcrafted herbs makes for a more delicious, health-giving tea.

BE AN INFORMED TEA DRINKER

When you think you've found a reputable brand of herbal tea, don't be afraid to ask the makers for information on their product. Read labels on the packages carefully and be conscious of environmentally friendly packaging.

I should point out that there is a difference between 'organic' and 'certified organic'. To label a tea 'certified organic', the tea must be strictly tested and conform to the criteria of a certification agency such as the Organic Growers Association or the National Association for Sustainable Agriculture Australia (NASAA). This is a rigorous and involved procedure, and not all tea manufacturers have the resources to undergo it. Many teas are labelled 'organic' because they are indeed cultivated without pesticides and other chemical additives, but they are not certified as such.

Cultivated, or non-organic, teas can still be of excellent quality. Many of these teas are cultivated in a similar fashion to organic teas, using herbs with a high level of active ingredients and produced to high standards. They simply may not carry the label 'organic', for reasons I have just mentioned. Always look for a reputable company.

Packaging for freshness

The packaging of loose-leaf herbal teas is crucial to maintaining its freshness and preserving its active ingredients. Herbs are a volatile product. They need to be stored, consumed and maintained as a fresh food. Just as fresh orange juice should be drunk immediately or soon after it has been made, similarly so should herbal teas be enjoyed. While herbal tea leaves can be reused for a second or third cup, they should not be left damp for longer than a few hours, and they should then not be recycled for further use (except on your garden beds or indoor plants).

Careful packaging is essential, especially for preservative-free organic and wildcrafted teas. Look for vacuum-packed or nitrogen-flushed teas. Both methods remove oxygen and moisture from the package, preventing its deterioration while sealed.

All herbal teas should be kept away from light and heat. However, when opened, organic herbal teas must be stored in an airtight container in the refrigerator, or at or below twelve degrees Celsius.

Finding a high-quality herbal tea will involve much trial and error. Keep these points in mind and be led by your taste. Is the tea full-bodied in flavour and aroma? Does it taste pure and clean? How does the tea make you *feel*? Does it soothe or invigorate you? Is it a pleasure to make and drink?

TIPS FOR CHOOSING QUALITY TEAS:

- *choose loose-leaf tea instead of teabags for its therapeutic properties, and its superior quality and taste*
- *experiment with different teas and manufacturers to find a tea that has a strong aroma, a lot of colour and full-bodied flavour*
- *always choose organic, wildcrafted or high-quality cultivated loose-leaf tea*
- *look for vacuum-packaged or nitrogen-flushed loose-leaf tea, which ensures tea remains fresh without the need for pesticides, preservatives and additives.*

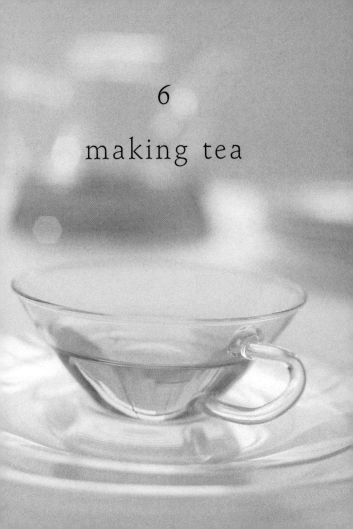

6

making tea

We all love – and need – to have our senses aroused. It's what makes us alive, what makes us human. Food, drink, art, film, clothing, sex, conversation, sport, music, dance, meditation – they awaken and captivate our sense of sight, touch, taste, smell and sound.

Consider the sensuality of drinking a glass of wine. After having carefully chosen the wine, you will have removed the cork and been immediately enticed by the first scent. You will have selected a glass specifically to complement the type of wine and indeed the occasion. You will have savoured the sound of the wine tickling the glass as it was poured. The colour will have caught your eye too: glistening and light, or smooth and rich. And then there is that lovely aroma again. All this and you haven't yet tasted the wine!

In the same way, the beauty and sensuality of loose-leaf herbal teas can be captured in the ritual of herbal tea making. This should come as no surprise. After all, the endless shapes, colours, textures and aromas of flowers and plants have always been a source of inspiration, relaxation and joy. The potpourri of loose leaves, flowers and berries that make a herbal tea blend brings the enjoyment of plants directly into our lives – and into our bodies.

The ritual of herbal tea making

When making your next cup of herbal tea, awaken your senses and follow these simple steps:

Take the time to smell the aroma of the loose-leaf tea you have chosen. You will need only one heaped teaspoon per cup if you are using a one-cup pot or plunger. If you are making tea for more than one person, use considerably less. As a general rule, if you are making tea for six people, use three to four teaspoons; if making tea for eight people, use four to five teaspoons. (It is important to note that you may use the same leaves two or three times, as the essential oils and other therapeutic properties are continually released from the herbs. Simply top up the pot with more freshly boiled water. The taste will remain the same.)

Measuring your tea

Because of their shape, regular teaspoons often fail to collect every ingredient in a tea blend. Try using a measuring spoon or a caddy spoon that is equal to one teaspoon, as these spoons will hold the dry ingredients more effectively.

Choose a suitable teapot or plunger. Glass teapots or plungers show the beauty of a herbal tea blend which a porcelain or pottery teapot would hide. On a practical level, glass retains the heat well and does not taint the flavour. (To retain the heat in a porcelain or pottery teapot, fill it with boiling water first and let it stand for a few minutes. Discard the water and then make the tea as required.)

  Always use fresh water. If the water from your tap is odorous or chemical-tasting, use filtered water. The water must be freshly boiled – not over-boiled or simply hot. This will ensure that both the taste and the health-giving properties of the tea are enhanced.

  Pour the boiled water over the herbs and watch the tea infuse. Herbal teas containing flowers and buds are particularly hypnotic to watch when they come into contact with boiled water. The colours are accentuated, and the flowers and buds open and sway, much like marine life. This is where a glass teapot or plunger is essential.

  Herbal tea made from leaves and flowers should stand for approximately three to four minutes. If the tea contains berries and roots, it should stand for up to fifteen minutes. This additional time is necessary because boiling water seeps into the harder parts of the herbs more slowly, gradually penetrating the fibres and extracting the plant's flavours and medicinal substances.

Keep a herbal-only teapot

Regardless of what kind of teapot you choose, use it for making herbal teas only. This is so that the herbs do not take on the taste of other drinks such as black and green teas or even coffee.

If you are using a regular teapot, be sure to use a strainer to catch the leaves. You can return the leaves to the pot to make another cup or two. When the leaves are spent, scatter them in your garden or on the base of your indoor plants.

Ideally you should drink herbal teas warm or at room temperature – not boiling. This is because the flavours of the herbs are enhanced at a lower temperature. It is also in the interests of your long-term health to avoid drinking boiling-hot beverages, as they literally scald your insides! At the very least, let the tea cool a little before tasting. And take your time drinking it.

❧ To make iced herbal tea, make the tea as above and place in the refrigerator. Alternatively, you could use one teaspoon of tea to half a cup of boiling water and then add iced water or ice blocks. And don't forget to reuse your tea leaves.

There are many varieties of herbal tea. Some are brightly coloured; others are not. Some contain flowers and berries; others contain only leaves of varying textures. Some are highly pungent; others contain only a gentle fragrance. Try a few different ones. Whatever tea you choose, go slowly the next time you make yourself a cup of herbal tea. Let your senses develop. Enjoy every sip.

and finally...

There is still so much we do not know, so much we do not understand, about plants and their therapeutic potential. The twenty-first century will be an exciting time in which the empirical art of plant medicine will continue to merge with scientific studies of plants and their active ingredients. From such a sharing of knowledge we can already understand why simple plants like chamomile and red clover really heal, and we can use this knowledge to help improve our daily lives.

People are beginning to recognise that refined food products do not give them the sustained energy they need to maintain a busy lifestyle. Many are returning to the basic principles of good health and are enjoying natural foods, lots of rest and relaxation, and exercise. They are increasingly seeking plant medicine to help them recuperate, rebuild and re-energise.

There is a danger, though, that with concentrated forms of herbs such as tablets and tinctures being so readily available, many people will seek to prescribe for themselves. Herbal healing is holistic. Herbal remedies must be tailored to a person's unique constitution, specific needs and individual circumstances. It is important to obtain an overall consultation from a practitioner at least three times a year, and to follow any prescriptions carefully.

Herbal teas are a safe natural remedy and have long been tried and tested as effective forms of plant medicine. Tea is a wonderful medium through which the healing properties of plants can be carried into the body. Tea is social. Tea is delicious. Tea is healing. Tea will surprise you.

bibliography

Bone, Kerry, *Clinical Applications of Ayurvedic and Chinese Herbs: Monographs for the western herbal practitioner*, Phytotherapy Press, Queensland, 1996.

Bone, Kerry & Mills, Simon, *Principles and Practice of Phytotherapy*, Churchill Livingstone, Edinburgh, 1999.

Bone, Kerry (ed.), 'Antioxidant flavonoids reduce heart risk', *Mediherb Monitor*, no. 9, June 1994.

Bone, Kerry (ed.), 'Antioxidant plants generate interest', *Mediherb Monitor*, no. 8, March 1994.

Bone, Kerry (ed.), 'Two for Tea', *Mediherb Monitor*, no. 23, September 1997.

Craze, Richard, *Herbal Teas*, New Holland Publishers, New South Wales, 1998.

Grieve, Mrs M., *A Modern Herbal*, Tiger Books International, London, 1994.

Hoffmann, David, *The Herbal Handbook: A Users Guide to Medical Herbalism*, Healing Arts Press, Vermont, 1987.

Marshall Marcin, Marietta, *The Complete Book of Herbal Teas: Growing, Harvesting, Brewing*, Congdon & Weed, New York, 1983.

Messegue, Maurice, *Health Secrets of Plants and Herbs*, William Collins, London, 1979.

Mills, Simon, *A Dictionary of Modern Herbalism*, Thorsons Ltd, London, 1985.

Mitscher, Lester A., Ph.D. & Dolby, Victoria, *The Green Tea Book: China's Fountain of Youth*, Avery Publishing Group, New York 1998.

Nakachi, K. et al., 'Influence of drinking green tea on breast cancer malignancy among Japanese patients', *Cancer Research*, vol. 89, no. 3, March 1998, pp. 254–61.

NASAA, 'Processing Standards for Certified Organic Food and Fibre' (booklet), South Australia, 1996.

Nutrition Society of Australia (Sydney Group), 'Antioxidants in Food, The Next Generation: The Science and the Practice', 3 July 1997.

Perry, Sara, *The Book of Herbal Teas: A Guide to Gathering, Brewing and Drinking*, Chronicle Books, San Francisco, 1997.

Pettigrew, Jane, *The Tea Companion: A Connoisseur's Guide*, Penguin Books, Victoria, 1999.

Sach, Penelope, *On Tea and Healthy Living*, Allen & Unwin, New South Wales, 1995.

Slavin, Sara & Petzke, Karl, *Tea: Essence of the Leaf*, Chronicle Books, San Francisco, 1998.

Smith, Dr Edward, 'The Action of Tea and Alcohols Contrasted', *The London Medical Review*, April 1861.

Smith, William, *Wonders in Weeds*, Camelot Press, Southampton, 1977.

Whitten, Greg, *Herbal Harvest: Commercial organic production of quality dried herbs*, Bloomings Books, Victoria, 1999.

Willson, K.C. & Clifford, M.N. (eds), *Tea: Cultivation to Consumption*, Chapman & Hall, London, 1992.

index

index

index

detox
Penelope Sach

Are you tired all the time? Is your body letting you down?

Modern life can be taxing on body and spirit. Here, naturo-path and herbalist Penelope Sach reveals ten simple detoxes to help you regain your energy and vitality.

This essential handbook for healthy living will show you:

- easy three-day detoxes
- specific detoxes for the skin, food additives and alcohol
- a special detox for anxiety and stress
- how to reduce and eliminate toxins from your life

plus there's a healthy living program for ongoing good health after detoxing.

Gentle and rejuvenating, detox works.

natural woman
Penelope Sach

In our increasingly chemical world, here are simple, natural solutions to health issues that every woman faces.

Naturopath and herbalist Penelope Sach details the symptoms, prevention and treatment of common physical and emotional concerns, including:

- weight control
- fatigue and depression
- stress
- skin conditions
- insomnia
- hormonal changes and ageing.

With indispensable advice for taking control of your health, *Natural Woman* will help you to look and feel your very best.